Erythromelalgia

A Beginner's Quick Start Guide to Managing the Condition Through Diet and Other Natural Lifestyle Changes, With Sample Curated Recipes

copyright © 2022 Patrick Marshwell

All rights reserved No part of this book may be reproduced, or stored in a retrieval system, or transmitted in any form or by any means, electronic, mechanical, photocopying, recording, or otherwise, without express written permission of the publisher.

Disclaimer

By reading this disclaimer, you are accepting the terms of the disclaimer in full. If you disagree with this disclaimer, please do not read the guide.

All of the content within this guide is provided for informational and educational purposes only, and should not be accepted as independent medical or other professional advice. The author is not a doctor, physician, nurse, mental health provider, or registered nutritionist/dietician. Therefore, using and reading this guide does not establish any form of a physician-patient relationship.

Always consult with a physician or another qualified health provider with any issues or questions you might have regarding any sort of medical condition. Do not ever disregard any qualified professional medical advice or delay seeking that advice because of anything you have read in this guide. The information in this guide is not intended to be any sort of medical advice and should not be used in lieu of any medical advice by a licensed and qualified medical professional.

The information in this guide has been compiled from a variety of known sources. However, the author cannot attest to or guarantee the accuracy of each source and thus should not be held liable for any errors or omissions.

You acknowledge that the publisher of this guide will not be held liable for any loss or damage of any kind incurred as a result of this guide or the reliance on any information provided within this guide. You acknowledge and agree that you assume all risk and responsibility for any action you undertake in response to the information in this guide.

Using this guide does not guarantee any particular result (e.g., weight loss or a cure). By reading this guide, you acknowledge that there are no guarantees to any specific outcome or results you can expect.

All product names, diet plans, or names used in this guide are for identification purposes only and are the property of their respective owners. The use of these names does not imply endorsement. All other trademarks cited herein are the property of their respective owners.

Where applicable, this guide is not intended to be a substitute for the original work of this diet plan and is, at most, a supplement to the original work for this diet plan and never a direct substitute. This guide is a personal expression of the facts of that diet plan.

Where applicable, persons shown in the cover images are stock photography models and the publisher has obtained the rights to use the images through license agreements with third-party stock image companies.

Table of Contents

Introduction	7
What Are the Two Primary Types of Erythromelalgia?	9
What Causes Erythromelalgia	11
What Are the Symptoms of Erythromelalgia	14
What Triggers Erythromelalgia?	16
What Are the Medical Treatments for Erythromelalgia?	18
What Are the Natural Treatments for Erythromelalgia?	21
Managing Erythromelalgia Through Lifestyle Changes	24
Managing Erythromelalgia Through Diet and Nutrition	26
Foods to Eat	26
Foods to Avoid	28
Sample Recipes	31
Baked Flounder	32
Salmon with Avocados and Brussels Sprouts	33
Asian-Themed Macrobiotic Bowl	35
Chicken Salad	37
Baked Salmon	38
Asian Zucchini Salad	39
Low FODMAP Burger	40
Stir-Fried Cabbage and Apples	41
Asparagus and Greens Salad with Tahini and Poppy Seed Dressing	42
Stir-Fried Cabbage and Apples	43
Roasted Chicken Thighs	44
Arugula and Mushroom Salad	45
Cauliflower and Mushroom Bake	46
Fresh Asparagus Salad	47
Detox Bowl	49

Managing Erythromelalgia Through Home Remedies   **51**
Conclusion   **54**
References and Helpful Links   **56**

Introduction

Erythromelalgia is a rare condition that typically affects the extremities, causing episodes of burning pain and redness. The condition is often associated with increased blood flow and temperature changes in the affected area. In some cases, erythromelalgia can also cause numbness or tingling.

The exact cause of erythromelalgia is unknown, but it is believed to be the result of abnormal blood vessel function. This may be due to an underlying condition such as diabetes, or it may be a primary condition.

There are two primary types of erythromelalgia, primary and secondary. Primary erythromelalgia is thought to be caused by an abnormality in the vascular system, while secondary erythromelalgia can be caused by a variety of underlying conditions, including diabetes, gout, and neuropathy.

There is no cure for erythromelalgia, but there are treatments available to help relieve the symptoms. In some cases, the condition may go into remission on its own.

Dietary and lifestyle changes can often help to lessen the severity of erythromelalgia symptoms. Avoiding triggers, such as heat, cold, or stress, can be helpful. Eating a healthy diet and maintaining a healthy weight is also important.

Natural remedies such as herbs and supplements may also help to relieve symptoms of erythromelalgia. Some people find relief with topical treatments such as capsaicin cream.

In this quick start guide, we will discuss the following in detail:

- What are the two primary types of erythromelalgia?
- What causes erythromelalgia?
- What are the symptoms of erythromelalgia?
- What triggers erythromelalgia?
- What are the medical treatments for erythromelalgia?
- How to treat erythromelalgia using natural remedies?
- Managing erythromelalgia through lifestyle changes
- Managing erythromelalgia through diet

Be sure to talk to your doctor before trying any natural remedies, as some may interact with medications you are taking or have other side effects.

What Are the Two Primary Types of Erythromelalgia?

There are two types of erythromelalgia: primary and secondary.

- *Primary erythromelalgia:* Primary erythromelalgia may appear to occur randomly for unknown reasons (sporadically) or rarely (in approximately 5% of cases) and may be familial. The exact cause of primary erythromelalgia is not known. However, it is thought to be related to problems with the nervous system that cause the body to overreact to stimuli (such as heat or touch) and dilate blood vessels excessively. This results in increased blood flow and warmth in the affected area.

- *Secondary erythromelalgia:* Secondary erythromelalgia is associated with an underlying cause, such as vascular abnormalities, inherited erythrocytosis syndromes, or medications. Secondary erythromelalgia is often caused by an underlying condition that results in abnormal blood vessels or changes in blood cells. In some cases, the cause of secondary erythromelalgia is not known.

Erythromelalgia can be a chronic (long-term) condition that can worsen over time. The pain associated with erythromelalgia can range from mild to severe and can interfere with daily activities. There is no cure for erythromelalgia, but treatments are available to help relieve symptoms.

What Causes Erythromelalgia

Depending on the type of erythromelalgia, different factors may be involved in its development.

Primary Erythromelalgia
- *Sporadic:* The cause of sporadic primary erythromelalgia is unknown. However, it is thought to be related to problems with the nervous system that cause the body to overreact to stimuli (such as heat or touch) and dilate blood vessels excessively. This results in increased blood flow and warmth in the affected area.

- *Familial:* Familial primary erythromelalgia is an inherited condition that is passed down from generation to generation in families. The exact cause of familial primary erythromelalgia is unknown, but it is thought to be related to problems with the nervous system that cause the body to overreact to stimuli (such as heat or touch) and dilate blood vessels excessively. This results in increased blood flow and warmth in the affected area.

Secondary Erythromelalgia

Secondary erythromelalgia can be caused by a variety of diseases, including:

- ***Fabry's disease:*** Fabry's disease is an inherited condition that causes a build-up of a fatty substance called gangliosides in the body. This build-up can damage blood vessels and nerves, resulting in erythromelalgia.

- ***Myeloproliferative disorders:*** Myeloproliferative disorders are conditions that cause the bone marrow to produce too many red blood cells. This can lead to an increase in blood viscosity (thickness), which can damage blood vessels and nerves, resulting in erythromelalgia.

- ***Autoimmune disorders:*** Autoimmune disorders occur when the body's immune system attacks and damages healthy tissues. This can lead to inflammation, which can damage blood vessels and nerves, resulting in erythromelalgia.

- ***Small fiber peripheral neuropathy:*** Small fiber peripheral neuropathy is a condition that results in damage to the small nerves in the arms and legs. This can cause pain, numbness, and tingling in the affected area. In some cases, small fiber peripheral neuropathy can also damage blood vessels, resulting in erythromelalgia.

- ***Mercury and mushroom poisoning:*** Mercury and mushroom poisoning can both cause erythromelalgia. Mercury poisoning can damage blood vessels and nerves, while mushroom poisoning can cause an immune reaction that leads to inflammation and damage to blood vessels.

- ***Use of certain medications:*** Some medications, such as beta-blockers, can cause erythromelalgia. This is thought to be because these medications can block the action of norepinephrine, a hormone that helps regulate blood vessel constriction.

- ***Hypercholesterolemia:*** Hypercholesterolemia is a condition that occurs when there is too much cholesterol in the blood. This can damage blood vessels and nerves, resulting in erythromelalgia.

What Are the Symptoms of Erythromelalgia

The symptoms of erythromelalgia can vary from person to person. In some cases, the symptoms are mild and only occur occasionally. In other cases, the symptoms are severe and may occur daily. If you experience any of the following symptoms, you should seek medical attention immediately.

- *Burning pain:* The most common symptom is burning pain that is felt in the hands, feet, or both. The pain is often described as a "pins and needles" sensation or as if the affected area is "on fire." The pain can range from mild to severe and can be intermittent or constant.

- *Skin redness:* One symptom of erythromelalgia is skin redness. The skin may appear reddish or flushed, and it may feel warm to the touch. The redness typically affects the hands and feet, but it can also affect the arms and legs. In some cases, the redness may spread to the trunk and other parts of the body. The redness is often accompanied by a burning or tingling sensation.

- *Numbness:* One symptom of erythromelalgia is numbness. This can be caused by inflammation and swelling reducing blood flow to the extremities. The reduced blood flow results in the nerves not getting enough oxygen, which causes them to malfunction and produce the sensation of numbness. In some cases, the reduced blood flow can also cause tissue damage. If you experience numbness in your extremities, it is important to seek medical help as soon as possible.

- *Changes in skin color:* A symptom of erythromelalgia, changes in skin color can be an early sign that something is wrong. The condition is caused by a problem with the blood vessels and nervous system, which results in increased blood flow to the extremities. This increased blood flow can cause the skin to appear reddish or flushed. In some cases, the skin may also feel warm to the touch.

What Triggers Erythromelalgia?

Several things can trigger erythromelalgia, including:

- *Heat:* People with erythromelalgia may have an increased sensitivity to heat due to alterations in their skin barrier function. This means that they may be more susceptible to discomfort or pain when exposed to warm temperatures. People with erythromelalgia often avoid hot weather and take measures to keep their skin cool, such as wearing loose-fitting clothing and using cooling devices.

- *Exercise:* Exercise can trigger erythromelalgia attacks. This is because exercise increases blood flow to the muscles, and in people with erythromelalgia, this increased blood flow can trigger an attack.

- *Stress:* Stress can also trigger erythromelalgia. This is thought to be because stress can increase blood flow and adrenaline levels, both of which can trigger an erythromelalgia attack.

- ***Diet:*** In some cases, erythromelalgia may be triggered by certain foods or beverages. Spicy food, chocolate, caffeine, and alcohol are all known to trigger erythromelalgia attacks in some people. If you suspect that certain foods are triggering your erythromelalgia attacks, it may be helpful to avoid these triggers or to eat them in moderation. You should also talk to your doctor about other potential treatment options for erythromelalgia.

These triggers can cause erythromelalgia attacks, which can last for a few minutes to a few hours. In some cases, erythromelalgia attacks can also last for days or weeks.

What Are the Medical Treatments for Erythromelalgia?

There is no cure for erythromelalgia, but there are treatments that can help relieve the symptoms.

- *Pain medications:* Pain medications, such as NSAIDs, can help to relieve the pain associated with erythromelalgia. NSAIDs work by reducing inflammation and swelling. They are available over-the-counter or on prescription. Side effects may include gastrointestinal upset, such as nausea and vomiting. In some cases, NSAIDs may also cause gastrointestinal bleeding. For these reasons, it is important to work with a doctor to determine the best course of treatment for erythromelalgia.

- *Antidepressants:* Antidepressants are commonly used to treat the pain associated with erythromelalgia. Tricyclic antidepressants, in particular, are effective in relieving the burning and throbbing sensations associated with the condition.

The mechanism by which tricyclic antidepressants provide pain relief is not fully understood. It is thought that they work by reducing the sensitivity of pain receptors. In addition to providing pain relief, tricyclic antidepressants can also help to improve mood and sleep quality. As a result, they are often an important part of treatment for erythromelalgia.

- *Calcium channel blockers:* Calcium channel blockers are a type of medication that is commonly used to treat high blood pressure and other cardiovascular conditions. By blocking the calcium channels in the body, these drugs help to improve blood flow and reduce inflammation. Calcium channel blockers are also sometimes used to treat other conditions, such as migraines and Raynaud's disease.

While these medications are generally safe and effective, they can cause side effects such as dizziness, headache, and nausea. Therefore, it is important to speak with a healthcare provider before starting any new medication.

- *Systemic corticosteroids:* Systemic corticosteroids are effective in reducing inflammation caused by erythromelalgia. These corticosteroids work by binding to receptors in the body to reduce inflammation. Prednisone is one type of systemic corticosteroid that is often used to treat erythromelalgia.

This medication can be taken orally or injected into the affected area. Systemic corticosteroids are typically well tolerated, but they can cause side effects such as weight gain, osteoporosis, and cataracts. When used correctly, however, they can be an effective treatment for erythromelalgia.

- *Surgery:* In severe cases of erythromelalgia, surgery may be necessary to remove damaged nerves or blood vessels. This type of surgery is typically performed by a neurologist or a vascular surgeon. The goal of surgery is to relieve pain and improve blood flow to the affected extremity. Surgery is usually only considered for people who have not responded to other treatments, such as medication or physical therapy. The risks and benefits of surgery should be discussed with a doctor before making a decision.

What Are the Natural Treatments for Erythromelalgia?

Several natural treatments can help relieve the symptoms of erythromelalgia.

- *Diet:* There is no cure for erythromelalgia, but there are some natural treatments that can help to reduce symptoms. One of the most important things you can do is to eat a healthy diet. Anti-inflammatory foods, such as omega-3 fatty acids, can help to reduce inflammation and improve blood flow.

  In addition, it's important to stay hydrated and avoid trigger foods or drinks, such as caffeine and alcohol. If you're struggling with erythromelalgia, talk to your doctor about a natural treatment plan that can help you find relief.

- *Supplements:* Several supplements can help improve blood flow and reduce inflammation. These include fish oil, ginger, ginkgo Biloba, and garlic. Fish oil is a rich source of omega-3 fatty acids, which have anti-inflammatory properties. Ginger is a common kitchen spice that's also been shown to reduce inflammation. Ginkgo Biloba is an herb that's been used for centuries to improve circulation. Garlic is another common ingredient that has anti-inflammatory properties.

These supplements can be taken orally or applied topically to the affected areas. If you're considering using any of these supplements, it's important to speak with your doctor first.

- *Exercise:* Exercise can help improve blood flow and reduce inflammation. It can also help to increase endorphins, which are natural painkillers. In addition, exercise can help to improve sleep and reduce stress, both of which can worsen erythromelalgia symptoms. If you have erythromelalgia, talk to your doctor about an exercise plan that is right for you.

- *Stress reduction:* Reducing stress can be an effective natural treatment for erythromelalgia. Stress can worsen the symptoms of erythromelalgia by constricting blood vessels and increasing inflammation. Stress-reduction techniques, such as meditation and yoga, can help improve blood flow and reduce inflammation.

- ***Acupuncture:*** By stimulating specific points in the body, acupuncture can help to restore the flow of qi and improve blood circulation. In addition, acupuncture can help to reduce inflammation and pain. A course of treatment typically consists of six to twelve sessions, and most patients report significant improvement after just a few treatments. If you are suffering from erythromelalgia, consider giving acupuncture a try.

Erythromelalgia is a condition that can be painful and debilitating. However, some treatments can help relieve the symptoms. by following a healthy diet, taking supplements, and reducing stress, you can help improve your erythromelalgia.

If you think you may have erythromelalgia, make an appointment with your doctor. They can help you find the best treatment for your symptoms.

Managing Erythromelalgia Through Lifestyle Changes

Living with erythromelalgia can be difficult, but there are some lifestyle changes you can make to help manage your symptoms.

- *Diet:* One way to manage erythromelalgia is to avoid trigger foods. Common trigger foods include spicy foods, caffeine, alcohol, and chocolate. If you have erythromelalgia, you may also want to avoid eating large meals or eating late at night. Eating smaller, more frequent meals throughout the day can help to reduce symptoms. It is also important to stay hydrated by drinking plenty of fluids.

- *Exercise:* Exercise is another important part of managing erythromelalgia. Exercise can improve blood circulation and help to reduce pain and swelling. However, it is important to avoid overheating, as this can trigger erythromelalgia flares. If you have erythromelalgia, be sure to dress in loose-fitting clothes and take breaks often when working out.

- ***Stress reduction:*** Stress can also exacerbate erythromelalgia symptoms, so it is important to find ways to relax and de-stress. Meditation, yoga, and deep breathing exercises can all help to reduce stress levels. In addition, try to get regular massages or take warm baths before bedtime. By following these tips, you can help to manage your erythromelalgia and live a more comfortable life.

Changing your lifestyle can be difficult, but it can help you manage your erythromelalgia. Talk to your doctor about what changes might be best for you.

Managing Erythromelalgia Through Diet and Nutrition

Foods to Eat

There are a few things you can do dietary-wise to help manage erythromelalgia. Eating a healthy diet is always important for overall health, but it can be especially helpful for managing erythromelalgia.

- *Vitamin B:* People suffering from erythromelalgia should make sure to consume foods that are high in vitamin B. This is because vitamin B is important for maintaining healthy nerves and blood vessels. Some good sources of vitamin B include meat, poultry, fish, eggs, dairy products, and leafy green vegetables.

- *Whole grains:* Eating foods that are high in fiber can help those who suffer from erythromelalgia, which is a disorder that causes extreme fatigue. Whole grains not only provide various nutrients that are necessary for healthy blood circulation, but they are also a good source of the fiber that our bodies need.

- ***Dairy:*** Patients diagnosed with erythromelalgia are frequently recommended to consume dairy products, as these items are an excellent source of calcium. Calcium is necessary for healthy bones and blood vessels, and it also has anti-inflammatory properties that might be helpful. In addition, erythromelalgia patients can benefit from the additional minerals, including vitamin D, that are found in dairy products.

- ***Vegetables:*** It is essential for persons who are afflicted with erythromelalgia to have a nutritious diet that is rich in fruits and vegetables in large quantities. Vegetables are an excellent source of many essential nutrients, including vitamins, minerals, and antioxidants, all of which can assist in the reduction of inflammation.

  Consuming a large number of vegetables regularly helps maintain healthy blood vessels, which plays a role in the prevention of erythromelalgia flares. Carrots, kale, spinach, and broccoli are some of the vegetables that are recommended for consumption by those who have erythromelalgia.

- ***Anti-inflammatory foods:*** The inflammation caused by erythromelalgia can be eased by eating certain foods, which can also help reduce inflammation overall. For instance, omega-3 fatty acids are well known for the anti-inflammatory characteristics that they possess. Nuts and seeds, as well as fatty seafood such as salmon and tuna, are good sources of these nutrients.

Ginger is another item that has the potential to help decrease inflammation. Recent research has indicated that this spice may be useful in treating erythromelalgia, one of the conditions that have been used throughout the years to treat a wide range of other conditions.

Last but not least, turmeric is another anti-inflammatory substance that might be useful for persons who suffer from erythromelalgia. The anti-inflammatory properties of this spice come from a component known as curcumin, which is found in this spice.

Foods to Avoid

There are a few things you can do dietary-wise to help manage erythromelalgia. One of these is to make sure you avoid these foods:

- *Sugar:* Sugar is a primary precipitating factor in erythromelalgia for the majority of affected individuals. Sugar consumption can lead to inflammation, which can make symptoms even more severe. It is also possible that it might bring on an episode of erythromelalgia in certain people. Because of this, persons who have erythromelalgia frequently need to limit the amount of sugar they consume.

- *Trans fats:* Trans fats are found in many processed foods and have been linked to an increased risk of erythromelalgia. A diet high in trans fats can worsen erythromelalgia symptoms and may even trigger the condition. Avoidance of trans fats may help improve erythromelalgia symptoms and prevent the condition from developing.

- *Alcohol:* Because it causes blood vessels to dilate, alcohol can make the symptoms of EM worse. This increases the amount of blood flowing to the afflicted region, which further amplifies the area's warmth and redness. Additionally, alcohol can cause the body to become dehydrated, which can increase both pain and inflammation. If you have EM, it is in your best interest to abstain from alcohol completely.

- *Spicy Foods:* Many people with erythromelalgia find that their symptoms are made worse by spicy foods. Capsaicin, the compound that gives chili peppers their heat, is known to trigger erythromelalgia flare-ups in some people. If you have erythromelalgia, you may want to avoid eating spicy foods or be careful to eat them in moderation. You should also talk to your doctor about ways to manage your symptoms and minimize flare-ups.

- *Garlic:* Garlic contains a compound called allicin, which can dilate blood vessels and increase blood flow. For people with erythromelalgia, this can cause intense burning pain. If you think that garlic may be worsening your erythromelalgia symptoms, talk to your doctor about avoiding garlic or other potential triggers.

Eating a healthy diet is important for managing erythromelalgia. Certain foods, such as sugar, trans fats, and processed foods, can worsen erythromelalgia symptoms. Eat anti-inflammatory foods, such as omega-3 fatty acids, and avoid foods that can worsen symptoms.

Sample Recipes

Baked Flounder

Ingredients:

- 1 lb. flounder, fileted
- 1/4 tsp. salt
- 1 cup halved red grapes
- 1 tbsp. extra-virgin olive oil
- 2 tbsp. parsley, chopped finely
- 1 tbsp. lemon juice
- 1 cup almonds, chopped and toasted
- freshly ground black pepper, to taste

Instructions:

1. Preheat the oven to 375°F.
2. Place fish on a sheet tray. Season with olive oil, salt, and pepper.
3. Combine the almonds, grapes, lemon juice, parsley, 1-1/2 tsp. of olive oil, 1/8 tsp of salt, and black pepper in a bowl.
4. Bake the fish for about 3 minutes.
5. Flip the fish and return to the oven.
6. Bake for another 3 minutes, or until the fish is starting to flake, while the center is still translucent. Don't overcook.
7. Serve immediately, topped with the grape mixture.

Salmon with Avocados and Brussels Sprouts

Ingredients:

- 2 lbs. of salmon filet, divided into 4 pieces
- 1 tsp. ground cumin
- 1 tsp. onion powder
- Himalayan sea salt
- black pepper, freshly grounded

Avocado sauce:

- 2 chopped avocados
- 1 lime, squeezed for the juice
- 1 tbsp. extra-virgin olive oil
- 1 tbsp. fresh minced cilantro
- 1 diced small red onion
- Himalayan sea salt to taste
- black pepper, freshly grounded

Brussels sprout:

- 3 lbs. of Brussels sprout
- 1/2 cup raw honey
- 1/2 cup balsamic vinegar
- 1/2 cup melted coconut oil
- 1 cup dried cranberries
- Himalayan sea salt to taste
- black pepper, freshly grounded

Instructions:

To make the salmon and avocado sauce:

1. Combine cumin, onion, seasoned with salt and pepper. Mix well before dry rubbing on the salmon.
2. Place the salmon in the fridge for 30 minutes.
3. Preheat the grill.
4. In a bowl, mash avocado until the texture becomes smooth. Pour in all the remaining ingredients and mix thoroughly.
5. Grill salmon for 5 minutes on each side or until cooked.
6. Drizzle avocado on cooked salmon.

To make the Brussel Sprout:

1. Preheat the oven to 375℉.
2. Mix Brussels sprouts with coconut oil. Season with salt and pepper.
3. Place vegetables on a baking sheet and roast for about 30 minutes.
4. In a separate pan, combine vinegar and honey.
5. Simmer in slow heat until it boils and thickens.
6. Drizzle them on top of the Brussels Sprouts.
7. Serve with the salmon.

Asian-Themed Macrobiotic Bowl

Ingredients:

- 2 cups cooked quinoa
- 4 carrots
- 1 package of smoked tofu
- 1 tbsp. nutritional yeast
- 2 tbsp. coconut aminos
- 4 tbsp. sunflower sprouts
- 2 tbsp. fermented vegetables
- 1 cup of shiitake mushrooms
- 1 avocado
- 2 tbsp. hemp seeds
- 2-3 cooked beets
- coconut oil cooking spray

Dressing:

- 2 tbsp. miso paste
- 1 tbsp. tahini
- 1 tbsp. olive oil
- 1/2 lime, juiced
- 3 tbsp. water

Instructions:

1. Roast the carrots in the oven at 400°F for 30-40 minutes.

2. Wash the vegetables, trim, and spray them with coconut oil.
3. Add them in the oven. When they are cooked, set aside till you are ready to assemble the Buddha bowl.
4. Make the dressing by combining all of the ingredients in a medium-size bowl. If the dressing appears lumpy, add more water.
5. To build the bowl, put the quinoa on the bottom and then arrange the vegetables on top.
6. Sprinkle the bowls with hemp seeds and drizzle the dressing over top.
7. Now serve and enjoy!

Chicken Salad

Ingredients:

- 1 small can premium chunk chicken breast packed in water
- 1 stalk celery, large, finely chopped
- 1/4 cup reduced-fat mayonnaise
- 4 romaine leaves or red leaf lettuce, washed and trimmed
- 8 pcs. cherry tomatoes or 1 ripe tomato, quartered
- 1 cucumber, small and sliced thinly

Instructions:

1. Drain canned chicken and transfer to a bowl.
2. Put in celery and mayonnaise.
3. Mix lightly. Don't crush the chicken.
4. In a separate shallow bowl, place the lettuce neatly.
5. Add the chicken salad in the middle
6. Add tomatoes and cucumber slices to the plate.
7. Refrigerate before serving, cover with plastic wrap.

Baked Salmon

Ingredients:

- 2 salmon filets
- 6 cups of fresh spinach
- 2 tsp. coconut oil
- 1/4 tsp. turmeric
- lemon juice
- salt
- pepper

Instructions:

1. Preheat the oven to 400°F.
2. Line a baking dish with parchment paper.
3. Marinate salmon filets in lemon juice, coconut oil, turmeric, salt, and pepper.
4. Let it sit for a few minutes. This may also be done the night before to help the juices and flavor get into the salmon.
5. Once the oven is ready, bake the salmon for 15 minutes.
6. Add spinach and cook until ready. Season with salt and pepper to taste.
7. Take salmon out of the oven and put spinach beside it.
8. Serve and enjoy.

Asian Zucchini Salad

Ingredients:

- 1 medium zucchini, sliced thinly into spirals
- 1/3 cup rice vinegar
- 3/4 cup avocado oil
- 1 cup sunflower seeds, shells removed
- 1 lb. cabbage, shredded
- 1 tsp. stevia drops
- 1 cup almonds, sliced

Instructions:

1. Cut the zucchini spirals into smaller parts. Set aside.
2. Put almonds, sunflower seeds, and cabbage in a large bowl. Combine the ingredients well.
3. Add zucchini to the mixture.
4. In a small bowl, mix vinegar, stevia, and oil using a whisk or fork.
5. Pour the vinegar mixture all over the zucchini mixture. Toss well. Make sure everything is covered with the dressing.
6. Refrigerate for 2 hours before serving.

Low FODMAP Burger

Ingredients:

- 1-1/4 lbs. ground pork
- 1/2 tsp. salt
- 1/2 tsp. white pepper
- 1/2 tsp. ground nutmeg
- 1/2 tsp. caraway seeds
- 1/2 tsp. ground ginger

Instructions:

1. Preheat the grill then prepare the patty.
2. Using a small mixing bowl, stir together the salt, pepper, nutmeg, and ginger until fully combined.
3. Place the ground in a large mixing bowl and add the spice mixture.
4. Mix thoroughly until spices are evenly distributed to the pork.
5. Make round, flat burger patties using the palm of your hands.
6. Grill the patties and serve with gluten-free buns and mustard sauce.

Stir-Fried Cabbage and Apples

Ingredients:

- 1 shallot, thinly sliced
- 1/2 apple, cut into cubes
- 1/4 savoy cabbage, sliced thinly into strips
- 3–4 radishes, sliced thinly
- 1/2–1 tsp. coconut oil
- salt, to taste

Instructions:

1. Pour some coconut oil into a wok.
2. Add shallot and cook until translucent.
3. Add the cabbage, radish, and apples to the wok.
4. Stir-fry for about 5 minutes. Don't overcook.
5. Add salt to taste.
6. Serve while warm.

Asparagus and Greens Salad with Tahini and Poppy Seed Dressing

Ingredients:

- 10 to 12 asparagus stalks, washed well and sliced into ribbons
- 5 radishes, washed well, and sliced thinly
- 2 to 3 rainbow carrots, peeled and sliced thinly
- 1 handful wild spinach
- 1 small handful of microgreens, washed well
- 1 small handful of sunflower greens, washed well
- optional: few pieces of chive blossoms

For the dressing:

- 2 tbsp. tahini
- 1 tbsp. poppy seeds
- 1 tbsp. extra-virgin olive oil
- salt
- pepper

Instructions:

1. For the dressing, whisk ingredients together in a small bowl.
2. In a separate bowl, toss salad ingredients in the mixture.
3. Drizzle dressing on salad upon serving.

Stir-Fried Cabbage and Apples

Ingredients:

- 1 shallot, thinly sliced
- 1/2 apple, cut into cubes
- 1/4 savoy cabbage, sliced thinly into strips
- 3–4 radishes, sliced thinly
- 1/2–1 tsp. coconut oil
- salt, to taste

Instructions:

1. Pour some coconut oil into a wok.
2. Add shallot and cook until translucent.
3. Add the cabbage, radish, and apples to the wok.
4. Stir-fry for about 5 minutes. Don't overcook.
5. Add salt to taste.
6. Serve while warm.

Roasted Chicken Thighs

Ingredients:

- 1 tbsp. avocado oil
- 1 pinch Himalayan pink salt
- 4 chicken thighs with skin
- 1 tsp. Primal Palate super gyro seasoning

Instructions:

1. Pour avocado oil over a medium-sized oven-safe pot.
2. Sauté over medium heat for 2 to 3 minutes or until the skins begin to brown.
3. Place the chicken in a large skillet over medium-high heat. Sear for about 2 to 3 minutes for each side, starting with the skin side.
4. Season generously with salt and Primal Palate Super Gyro seasoning.
5. Place the chicken in an oven preheated to 350°F.
6. Bake for one hour while covered.
7. Serve and enjoy.

Arugula and Mushroom Salad

Ingredients:

- 5 oz. arugula washed
- 1 lb. fresh mushrooms
- 1/4 tsp. shoyu
- 1/2 red onion
- 1 tbsp. olive oil
- 1 tbsp. mirin

For tofu cheese:

- 1/8 cup umeboshi vinegar
- 1/2 firm tofu

Instructions:

1. In a bowl, add the rinsed tofu. Crumble and pour in vinegar.
2. In a separate bowl add shoyu, red onions, salt, olive oil, and mirin. 3. Mix to combine.
3. Add in the arugula and toss to combine with the dressing.
4. Serve and enjoy.

Cauliflower and Mushroom Bake

Ingredients:

- 3 cups cauliflower florets
- 1 cup fresh mushroom, chopped
- 1/2 cup red onion, chopped
- 1/3 cup green onion, chopped
- 2 tsp. apple cider vinegar
- 2 tsp. lemon juice
- 1/2 tsp. salt
- 1/4 tsp. pepper
- 1 tbsp. olive oil

Instructions:

1. Preheat the oven to 350°F. Lightly grease a baking pan.
2. Combine red onion, cauliflower, olive oil, mushroom, apple cider vinegar, lemon juice, salt, and pepper in a bowl. Mix well.
3. Pour the mixture into the greased baking pan.
4. Place inside the oven and bake for 45 minutes. Stir.
5. When vegetables are golden brown and tender, remove from the oven.
6. Garnish with green onions. Serve and enjoy.

Fresh Asparagus Salad

Ingredients:

- 1/3 cup of hazelnuts
- 4 cups arugula
- 1 tsp. ground pepper
- 4 tsp. lemon juice
- 2 tbsp. sea salt
- virgin olive oil
- 2 lbs. asparagus

Instructions:

1. Preheat the oven to 400°F.
2. Place hazelnuts on a baking tray with parchment paper. Place in the oven for 7 minutes.
3. Transfer hazelnuts to a plate. Optionally, to remove the skins, wrap the nuts in a towel and rub them vigorously.
4. Chop hazelnuts coarsely.
5. Remove the hard ends of the asparagus.
6. Place the stalks on the baking sheet you've used for the hazelnuts. Sprinkle 1 tbsp. olive oil and 1/2 tsp. of salt.
7. Bake for 8 minutes.
8. In a mixing bowl, combine pepper, salt, olive oil, and lemon juice. Mix well.

9. Place the arugula in a medium bowl. Drizzle ½ of the dressing over the veggies. Toss until everything is well coated.
10. Place arugula onto a platter.
11. Arrange asparagus on top. Sprinkle peeled hazelnuts on top.

Detox Bowl

Ingredients:

- 1/2 cup onion, diced
- 1-1/2 tbsp. olive oil or coconut oil
- 1 tbsp. ginger, grated
- 1 tsp. whole mustard seeds
- 1 tsp. turmeric
- 1/2 tsp. cumin
- 1/2 tsp. coriander
- 1/2 tsp. curry powder, add more for taste
- 3/4 tsp. kosher salt
- 1/4 lentils, soaked overnight
- 1/2 cup buckwheat, toasted or brown basmati rice, soaked
- 1-1/2 cup water
- 1 cup vegetable broth
- 2 cups vegetables, chopped such as broccoli, carrot, cauliflower, celery, a fennel bulb, and parsnips
- 2 tbsp. cilantro or Italian parsley, chopped
- lemon or lime, squeezed
- 1 tomato, diced

Instructions:

1. Heat up oil on a medium pot over medium-high heat.
2. Saute onion for about 2-3 minutes.

3. Lower heat to medium and add ginger to saute for a few minutes, or until it's fragrant and the color turns golden.
4. Add salt and pepper according to your taste. Stir and leave to toast for a few more minutes.
5. Put lentils and buckwheat or rice, followed by water, broth, and the remaining vegetables. Bring to a boil and cover.
6. Reduce heat to low and leave to simmer for about 20 minutes. Check every now and then for doneness.
7. Leave to cook for 5-10 minutes more if needed.
8. For porridge-like consistency, pour in more veggie broth.
9. Upon serving, top with tomato and cilantro or parsley. Dash with salt, pepper, and a choice of citrus. Drizzle olive oil if desired.

Managing Erythromelalgia Through Home Remedies

Several home remedies can help improve erythromelalgia symptoms.

- ***Cold compress:*** A person suffering from erythromelalgia may find relief from the associated pain and inflammation by applying a cold compress to the region that is afflicted by the condition. This is because cold temperatures assist to constrict blood vessels, which in turn decreases the amount of blood flow to the region, which in turn lessens the amount of inflammation. In addition, the pressure from the compress can aid to prevent pain signals from reaching the brain, which can be a beneficial effect.

    However, to prevent the compress from making direct contact with the affected region and causing additional irritation, it is essential to wrap it in a towel or another piece of fabric before applying it. It is recommended that the compress be applied for a period of 15 to 20 minutes at a time, many times each day.

- ***Warm bath:*** A warm bath is one of the most efficient treatments for lowering pain and increasing circulation, and there are very few other methods that come close. As a result of the heat of the water helping to dilate blood vessels and enhance blood flow, one may experience an instant reduction in pain as well as an improvement in muscular function.

   In addition, the warmth of the water can assist to relax tight muscles, which is another factor that contributes to the reduction of pain. Those who suffer from erythromelalgia may find that a relaxing soak in a hot bath provides great relief from the condition's symptoms.

- ***Massage:*** A reduction in discomfort and an increase in blood flow are two benefits that may be achieved by the application of massage to the afflicted region. In addition, rubbing the afflicted area can assist to promote the production of endorphins, which are chemicals in the body that have a natural analgesic effect.

   As a consequence of this, massaging the region that is afflicted by erythromelalgia is an efficient method for reducing pain and improving circulation in persons who suffer from erythromelalgia.

- ***Reducing stress:*** Even though erythromelalgia cannot be cured, there are treatments available that can help manage the illness and lessen its symptoms. One of the most efficient strategies is to lower one's stress levels. Because it causes blood vessels to constrict and raises inflammatory levels, stress can make erythromelalgia symptoms worse.

  However, stress-reduction strategies like yoga and meditation can assist to increase blood flow and reduce inflammation in the body. As a direct consequence of this, the procedures can be of great assistance to individuals who suffer from erythromelalgia.

In addition to conventional medical therapy, the use of home treatments for erythromelalgia may prove beneficial. However, home remedies are not intended to replace professional medical care in any way.

Conclusion

Erythromelalgia is a disorder that can be challenging to manage on a day-to-day basis. The discomfort may be crippling, and the itching sensation that never goes away can be extremely annoying. Although there is currently no cure for erythromelalgia, there are therapies that can assist to alleviate some of the condition's symptoms.

It's possible that some people with erythromelalgia can find relief from their discomfort and itching with over-the-counter treatments, while others will need medication that's only available by prescription.

Alterations to your way of life, such as those mentioned above, may also be of assistance in the management of your symptoms. Erythromelalgia symptoms can be improved by maintaining a healthy weight, getting regular exercise, and lowering stress levels. There are also some things you may do at home to assist, such as warm baths and cold compresses. If you have been diagnosed with erythromelalgia, you should discuss potential lifestyle adjustments with your attending physician.

Many persons with erythromelalgia can discover solutions to manage the symptoms of their disease and lead fulfilling lives despite the difficulties of living with the condition.

This article is meant solely for educational reasons and is not intended to serve as a replacement for professional medical advice or treatment. Please consult your primary care physician if you have any worries or queries regarding the state of your health.

References and Helpful Links

"An Overview of Erythromelalgia." Verywell Health, https://www.verywellhealth.com/erythromelalgia-overview-4582735. Accessed 24 Sept. 2022.

ePainAssist, Team. "What Is Erythromelalgia|Causes|Signs|Symptoms|Treatment|Surgery|Diet|Diagnosis." Epainassist, 16 May 2016, https://www.epainassist.com/vascular-disease/what-is-erythromelalgia.

"Erythromelalgia: Symptoms, Causes, Treatment." Cleveland Clinic, https://my.clevelandclinic.org/health/diseases/22752-erythromelalgia. Accessed 24 Sept. 2022.

Jha, Suman K., et al. "Erythromelalgia." StatPearls, StatPearls Publishing, 2022. PubMed, http://www.ncbi.nlm.nih.gov/books/NBK557787/.

Erythromelalgia is a rare condition that typically affects the extremities, causing episodes of burning pain and redness. The condition is often associated with increased blood flow and temperature changes in the affected area. In some cases, erythromelalgia can also cause numbness or tingling.

The exact cause of erythromelalgia is unknown, but it is believed to be the result of abnormal blood vessel function. This may be due to an underlying condition such as diabetes, or it may be a primary condition.

There are two primary types of erythromelalgia, primary and secondary. Primary erythromelalgia is thought to be caused by an abnormality in the vascular system, while secondary erythromelalgia can be caused by a variety of underlying conditions, including diabetes, gout, and neuropathy.

Natural remedies such as herbs and supplements may also help to relieve symptoms of erythromelalgia. Some people find relief with topical treatments such as capsaicin cream.

In this quick start guide, we will discuss the following in detail:
- What are the two primary types of erythromelalgia?
- What causes erythromelalgia?
- What are the symptoms of erythromelalgia?
- What triggers erythromelalgia?
- What are the medical treatments for erythromelalgia?
- How to treat erythromelalgia using natural remedies?
- Managing erythromelalgia through lifestyle changes.
- Managing erythromelalgia through diet.

A Beginner's 3-Week Step-by-Step Guide for Women, With Sample Curated Recipes and a Meal Plan

ECZEMA
Diet Plan

Stephanie Hinderock

www.ingramcontent.com/pod-product-compliance
Lightning Source LLC
LaVergne TN
LVHW012038060526
838201LV00061B/4662